what's a nice person like you doing sick?

what's a nice person like you doing sick?

paul e. parker, m.d.
with
david enlow

creation house
carol stream, illinois

© 1974 by Creation House. All rights reserved.
Published by Creation House,
499 Gundersen Drive, Carol Stream, Illinois 60187.
In Canada: Beacon Distributing Ltd.,
104 Consumers Drive, Whitby, Ontario L1N 5T3.

Illustrations by Darrell Wiskur.

Printed in the United States of America.

Biblical quotations are reprinted with permission
from the New American Standard Bible
© 1971 by the Lockman Foundation.

ISBN 0-88419-082-X

Library of Congress Catalog Card Number 74-82838

contents

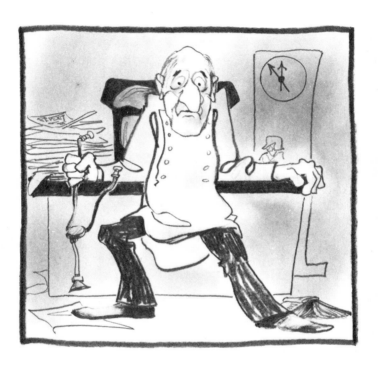

accepting my condition

1

Doctors, like mothers, simply aren't allowed to get sick.

Actually, I had been too busy even to think about it. Office and hospital rounds, plus occasional calls at odd times of the night, kept me going at a frantic pace. Sleep had become a cherished luxury.

Early one morning I awoke with a different feeling than usual. Slight fever, sore throat, runny nose—all the symptoms of a cold, or at worst, a light touch of the flu. Taking the usual precautions, I plodded along with my normal duties. But the second morning was no better, and the third was worse.

My mind went back a couple of weeks. I had been feeling tired and draggy and had a few small night sweats. It must have been just laziness or lack of physical activity, I thought. I had set several rows of hedge and had repaired the roof, all the time wondering why I felt so exhausted. Maybe I was coming down with the flu.

I hadn't suffered any serious illness since I was seven—some forty-six years earlier. But when my urine became dark, I checked it myself and found bile in it. That gave me a rather strange sensation, for I knew it could lead to anything from chronic liver deficiency to death (for about five percent in my age range).

I just *knew* it couldn't be me. (I began to understand in a new way just how my patients felt under similar circumstances. Right then and there I resolved to do better in anticipating their questions.)

The next morning I went over to the lab in my clinic and wrote out a requisition for a number of tests. I fully suspected hepatitis, and I knew that no medicine would treat it. The only answer was total bed rest.

I went up to my office waiting room, where doctors, nurses, and patients went purposefully about their business. My predicament puzzled me. They were all so busy; I felt embarrassed to say, "Could you work me in?" Finally I asked a colleague, "Do you think you would have time to look me over?"

Shortly, the nurse took me in, and after about two hours I had the confirming evidence. (Again, I realized the trauma most patients encounter simply by having to wait so long.)

My mind raised the usual questions. How would I adjust? Would the disease affect me the same way it had other adults I had known? Hepatitis is usually a disease of younger people; many adults suffer long or even die from it. What would happen to the family, with the breadwinner laid aside for a few months, or longer?

Had I known then what I know now, the feeling of frustration and dependence would not have been so severe. But such foresight, even though it might have eased my discomfort, quite likely would have reduced the value of lessons I needed to learn. I had heard that many of life's greatest lessons come in the crucible of pain and suffering. That had been a pious platitude; it was to become a ringing reality.

Every person, in his darkest hours, must have some base he can touch. Mine happened to be the Word of God, and the God of the Word. Early in my illness, I recalled the scriptural command, "In everything give thanks." Really? In *everything?* That's what it said, so I began to practice. But it didn't come easy.

"God, thank You for the hepatitis. I don't enjoy it; I don't like it, but there must be a purpose in it—Your purpose for me— so I thank You for it."

And so on, down the line: "God, thank You for the nausea; thank You for the severe headaches; thank You for the fever." But each new step of faith seemed traumatic.

One of the easiest and most natural things in the world to do when we are sick is to ask *why.* One of the hardest things in the world to do is to thank the Lord for our illness. But one road leads to defeat, the other to victory.

Actually, nothing about the nausea, the fever,

the headaches earned my appreciation. But somehow I knew my condition, as uncomfortable as it was, must be reconciled with certain plain-spoken portions of the Word of God.

I had planned to take my son to Explo '72 in Dallas. Billy Graham and Johnny Cash would participate before a hundred thousand young people in the Cotton Bowl. I was scheduled for two workshops myself. And I was planning to visit my aged parents in Tucson—a chance to meet my obligations as a son. *Why couldn't this illness have come three weeks later?* But the more I considered the situation, the more I realized I must be thankful for everything— even God's timing in my illness.

I really didn't have to know *why* the timing was this way—only to accept it as His. The same was true with every new experience of my illness. "God," I prayed, "thank You for helping me to see sickness from a patient's point of view."

There seemed no escaping the plain teaching of the Word. How could I get around Epheians 5:20, "Always giving thanks for all things . . ."? And why should I be expected to give thanks for *all* things? The answer came with another clear portion of the Word, "And we know that God causes all things to work together for good to those who love God, to those who are called according to His purpose" (Romans 8:28).

One is a direct command, the other a promise.

Add still one more promise, "To obey is better than sacrifice . . . ," and I realized I was inextricably bound. Scripture does not always make plain the *why* of its promises, but it does clearly state the intent—and the conditions; the same with commands. Though at first I felt phony and Pollyannish by praising when I didn't really feel like it, my obedience was counted for gain, for righteousness. And it was the key that unlocked the door of God's working in my life.

It wasn't easy, but I knew the road I must take. If the Word of God is true—and I certainly had no doubts about it—then I would have to acknowledge its promises and conditions and obey its commands in order to truly experience any degree of joy and victory.

Granted, you may experience the same thing I did—utter foolishness the first time I thanked God for physical suffering. But it wasn't long before the "foolishness" resulted in faith and triumph. The sickness, the suffering, the discomfort remained for an extended period, but an indescribable inner peace accomplished an "impossible" end result: *real joy.*

Simple logic forced me to accept the reasoning of the Word, even as I lay often with pain and discomfort. I had no problem accepting the promise of eternal life through faith in Jesus Christ. Should I not just as easily accept the promise that "God causes all things to work together for good to those who love God . . ."?

Learning to accept my condition was a major step in my restoration to health. Fighting my condition certainly would lead to nothing more than frustration and fearfulness. In the final analysis, it all boiled down to one simple question: *Would I believe God, or would I not?*

Strengthening one's faith is a vital part of this whole process, and I knew of no better way than to follow another scriptural suggestion: "Faith comes by hearing, and hearing by the word of Christ." A good concordance helped me immensely in finding passages on faith and healing. A regular reading of the Psalms did much to bolster my faith, for in the Psalmist we see a man who experienced many of the same fears and frustrations we face—and yet "a man after God's own heart."

But after reading these faith-strengthening passages, I still had to come back to the clearly defined promises and commands:

"Always giving thanks for all things . . . ."

"For we know that God causes all things to work together for good to those who love God, to those who are called according to His purpose."

"To obey is better than sacrifice."

Ultimately, I had to come to the realization and accept the fact that "God works in mysterious ways His wonders to perform." One of these mysterious ways is often illness. I found that accepting the premise that "God is not through with me yet" led to victory, if in that acceptance I included the matter of illness—in all its forms.

14

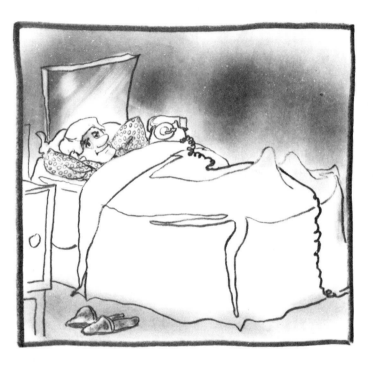

worry makes it worse

With almost every prolonged illness come twin specters: anxiety and depression. My case was no exception. But God did tell me what to do with these ogres.

First, I was not to feel guilty for having such intruders. It was a normal experience.

Second, I was to treat every experience of anxiety and depression as an *object*. At its first appearance I was to turn that object over to God Himself by a deliberate act of the will. Then I should remind Him that I was too weak and helpless to do anything about it. It was His problem now.

Thus turning the responsibility over to Him, I focused my attention heavenward rather than inward. I saw a remarkable thing take place. In a matter of hours, I realized that anxiety and depression had left. Peace reigned. But this was not a mechanical thing. Sometimes I had to turn the *object* over to Him as many as thirty times before any real, lasting peace came. But every experience of this kind accomplished one major purpose: it strengthened me physically and spiritually.

As I lay there day after day, it became quite

frustrating at times. Spring was coming on, and my wife would go out and work in the yard. I'd see the kids going off to school. All I could do was to lie in bed. "You have to stay quiet," I was reminded often by my doctor and my family.

A frightening thing happened about the fifth night. Some two or three hours past midnight, a loud knock at the back door roused me from a fitful, restless sleep. A panicky feeling enveloped me. I was not strong enough to take care of my own family. "Well, God," I prayed hurriedly, fervently, "You'll have to take care of them Yourself."

The police responded to my call in a matter of minutes. They searched, and I searched, but no one could be found. I did learn a new sense of dependence on the Lord, however.

One thing in particular helped alleviate the fears and worries that constantly threatened to engulf me. Friends sent me cards, letters, and books, and many called me by phone. All assured me of their prayers in my behalf. I saw a tremendous strength and unity in the Body of Christ, and it cheered and encouraged me. I learned anew the cohesiveness and interdependence of that Body. We all need each other.

One need not go all the way with the stress theory of sickness to appreciate the harmfulness of worry. That theory, of course, maintains that all sickness and disease stem from stress in one form or another. To accelerate that stress by hard-nosed worry can only complicate the situation.

My reaction to the onslaught of hepatitis was quite natural. The disease is characterized by weakness, often sheer exhaustion. As soon as supper was over, I was ready for sleep. Often I felt a gnawing pain in the pit of the stomach, not severe, but unpleasant and continuous. That lasted off and on for about a week or ten days. I knew that any medicine taken would have to be broken down by the liver, so it was really best not to take any, in spite of the pain.

Often during the night I would awaken with severe headaches. Add all of these things together and you can see why Satan comes in to capitalize on them with a vast barrage of temptations, thoughts, and suggestions. The very fact that they are so depressing makes one feel guilty.

Strangely, perhaps, another strong testing came when I began to feel better. I still had to stay in bed, which was tremendously burdensome and frustrating. Though my attention span was short, I didn't let this bother me. When I became tired of listening to medical tapes, I simply switched to reading books, listening to the radio, or watching television occasionally.

Later, when Tedd Seelye interviewed me on Radio Station WMBI, the voice of the Moody Bible Institute in Chicago, I learned there are many people who face this kind of problem—not just for ten or eleven weeks, but for a lifetime.

Later (in chapter 4) I want to suggest a few things that helped me and others.

I learned that one practice, in particular, knocks worry for a loop; that is the practice of praise—of thanking God in and for everything. Again, I found that difficult, even impossible at times. But it followed as plainly as night follows day that peace followed praise.

Not everyone responds to illness in the same way, nor to the varying degrees of illness, but this is not primarily what we are talking about here. The late prophet of God, Dr. A. W. Tozer, whose editorials, books, and preaching ministry have blessed and strengthened many thousands of people, used to say that he could never feel spiritual if he had a bad cold. Many of us respond similarly to weaknesses of the flesh.

But by faith we can learn to thwart the enemy of men's souls by refusing to fall into his favorite trap—worry. Dr. Tozer found a way around his problem, and you and I can do the same. He reminded himself that worry, despair, and discouragement were never sent by the Lord; hence they must be tools of the devil. On that basis, he refused to accept them. Again, I found it necessary to repeat this kind of exercise in faith many times.

This was not for Dr. Tozer, nor will it be for you, a once-for-all-time experience. The temptation to worry is as common as the temptation to any other—and *most* other—kinds of sin. We need to remind ourselves often:

temptation is not a sin; it is only in yielding to it that we fall into sin.

And even when the old nature wins out, as it almost inevitably must at times, we have a glorious way of escape. "If we confess our sins [including worry], He is faithful and righteous to forgive us our sins and to cleanse us from all unrighteousness" (I John 1:9).

The antidote for worry: praise.

In his helpful book *God Blessed Me with a Heart Attack*, Richard G. Dunwoody confessed he was "ashamed of the anxiety which I saw in my soul. Little children trust their parents for everything. They don't worry, their nerves are not taut and jaded with cares. They know mother and father will take care of them. They implicitly trust their parents—parents who are weak, limited, who sometimes fail. Yet we, as God's children, fail to trust Him who has all power and who never fails."

Not without good reason, Dr. John Edmund Haggai *(How to Win over Worry)* calls worry "Public Enemy No. 1." Worry causes heart trouble, high blood pressure, asthma, rheumatism, ulcers, colds, arthritis, migraine headaches, blindness, and many stomach disorders including ulcers, according to some specialists, and I would not argue with them.

One of Dr. Haggai's most meaningful reminders is this: "No one can pray and worry at the same time. 'Thou wilt keep him in perfect peace, whose mind is stayed on thee: because he trusteth in thee' (Isaiah 26:3)."

I found that delightfully true: when I met the conditions, I experienced the promised peace. Since worry only makes things worse, I counterattacked with prayer and praise. Victory is assured.

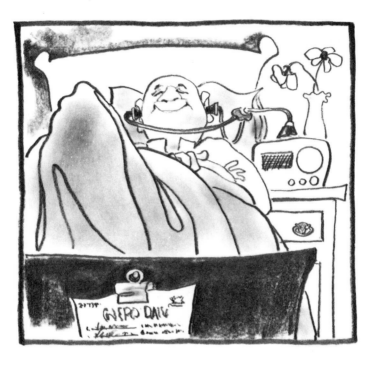

how to develop
a positive mental attitude

There is something good to be said about a positive attitude, and it comes right from the Word of God: "As a man thinketh in his heart, so is he" (Proverbs 23:7, King James Version).

It takes practice—constant practice, in fact a lifetime of it—to maintain this kind of attitude. But it is well worth the effort.

This does not mean that you and I are to bypass harsh reality. To properly cultivate this kind of attitude, we must be frank with ourselves and with God. When I faced my own physical dilemma, I learned to talk plainly in prayer. God knows all about me, anyway. Why not be frank with Him?

"God," I would pray, "I'm not real happy with what You're doing in my life just now, but I know You're doing the right thing. You've promised that 'all things work together for good to those who love God.' I believe You, so I thank You for this experience which is painful."

Having faced the problem squarely, I felt I now had the right to proceed with a positive attitude, knowing that my case was in the best possible hands. When our foundation is the Creator Himself, the Maker of the universe, the heavenly Father, our attitude truly is well-founded when it looks on the bright side of seemingly hopeless situations.

In recent years particularly, I have become greatly interested in the concept that much disease occurs because we have a lowered resistance. This comes about when we disregard God's natural laws by working harder than He intends us to do. I realized there had been a definite pattern that lowered my resistance. In the preceding weeks and months, I had had two major decisions to make, each involving some emotional stress.

One came when a colleague of mine went off to teach in Canada. He was one of my best friends, and I missed him greatly. A few weeks before he left I suddenly realized he wouldn't be here anymore; it was like losing a brother. How would we provide the medical care for his patients? Our schedules already overflowed with responsibilities. I found myself watching the daily census at the clinic: forty-seven patients in one day. Though I didn't like it, I had to rush in and out of rooms as I treated the patients.

Soon the inevitable happened: I became impatient. I was seeing more patients but enjoying it less. Pressure and frustration multiplied, and still we were not seeing all the patients. It became a real source of tension and anxiety. I even thought of leaving the clinic.

An offer to serve as a hospital medical director

brought about another major decision. Even after giving an affirmative answer, I had no real peace about it. I realized that my real satisfaction in medicine was in knowing people, so that I didn't mind treating flu, ordinary colds, and anything else as long as they were in the people I knew. If I took the hospital position, I would have to totally give up this relationship. I wouldn't see my friends any more.

The late Marion Wade, founder of ServiceMaster, for example. I always had looked forward to his visits. I had developed a real admiration for him, an enjoyment of our time together. I would be divorcing myself from a lot of friends.

There was nothing to do, of course, but to reconsider my previous decision. And when I finally gave up the hospital position, I had the added tension of a guilt complex—feeling perhaps I had let down my friend at the hospital.

Through all of this long period of indecision, anxiety, and uncertainty, my resistance was lowered. This may well explain why I came down with hepatitis. In some ways my attitude had not been right. I had not developed the ability to truly turn over my problems to the Lord. I had not learned to accept less from myself, to realize God is satisfied with my doing less than I think I have to be doing.

Sometimes there is a temptation in a doctor's life to want to feel needed by everyone. I learned that God doesn't want me to do everything. I had to rearrange my priorities and be satisfied with what God is satisfied with: *doing one thing at a time.*

A friend of mine said to me recently, "I feel so good; I have just resigned from eight boards." He had allowed his life to be overloaded with good things. We need to have faith in God's plan—His will—for our lives. We get brainwashed by the world in the matter of efficiency and accomplishments.

A friend of mine told me of once visiting C.S. Lewis' housekeeper. The servant commented that people would see Lewis walking by the hour and would look on him as "an old man wasting his time." What they didn't know was that from his walks and meditations would come some of Christendom's finest writings.

I learned not to program my schedule too tightly. There must be some gaps, some open time in the schedule. Unprogrammed time allows us to do some very valuable creative things. And all of this changes our attitude for the better.

Usually, none of us starts out with a right attitude. It is something that is developed, cultivated, nourished. When Richard G. Dunwoody went through his harrowing heart attack experience at the relatively young age of thirty-seven, his first reaction was rebellion, followed by resignation, then thanksgiving. But he knew the proper attitude to cultivate, which accounted for the overwhelming victory he experienced through it all.

I still find it one of the great mysteries of life, but the fact remains that each of us can genuinely help to create the kind of attitude we want to have. For example, I may begin the day feeling anything but joyful. But the Bible says, "Consider it all joy . . . ." By faith, I do that very thing—and the miracle takes place. Soon I begin to deeply feel the kind of joy I have determined to express.

It became clear to me that the same principle applies to other characteristics. On more than one occasion I have lacked real enthusiasm about beginning another day. But the Word of God says, "Whatever you do, do your work *heartily* . . . ." So in simple obedience I begin to practice being enthusiastic. Again, mysteriously, it is not very long before genuine enthusiasm envelops me.

In the matter of illness, serious or otherwise, I wanted first of all to maintain a strong faith in an all-wise Providence who has my life and all that concerns me in the hollow of His hand. I began to exercise that faith, ever so feebly at first, but then increasingly stronger as God honored the earnest effort to please Him.

In my illness, I wanted somehow to reflect honor to the Lord and at the same time radiate His love to others. This was not a natural procedure under such adverse circumstances, so I began to pray for the supernatural—His perfect peace that passes all understanding.

Against all evidence to the contrary, I tried to think that God was performing His best for me—His perfect will in my life. By faith I cultivated those positive thoughts and rejected the negative. When my condition was too weak to do battle against the intrusion of wrong thoughts, I still counted on God to fight my battle for me. And He did.

I have seen an anonymous prayer, displayed on desks, that describes the kind of attitude I would like to maintain at all times:

Slow me down, Lord! Ease the pounding of my heart by the quieting of my mind. Steady my hurried pace with a vision of the eternal reach of time. Give me, amid the confusion of the day, the calmness of the everlasting hills. Break the tensions of my nerves and muscles with the soothing music of the singing streams that live in my memory. Help me to know the magical, restoring power of sleep. Teach me the art of taking minute vacations—of slowing down to look at a flower, to chat with a friend, to pat a dog, to read a few lines from a good book. Remind me each day of the fable of the hare and the tortoise, that I may know that the race is not always to the swift; that there is more to life than increasing its speed. Let me look upwards into the branches of the towering oak and know that it grew great and strong because it grew slowly and well.

Slow me down, Lord, and inspire me to send my roots deep into the soil of life's enduring values that I may grow toward the stars of my greater destiny. In Jesus' name. Amen.

Untold numbers of people are watching your life and mine, whether on our sickbed or at the office. Our attitude under adversity will say more to them than anything else we can possibly say. May it speak of God's goodness in and through it all.

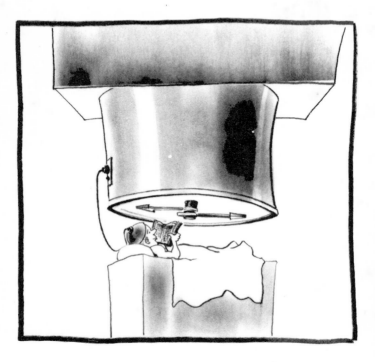

using time wisely

It was not just anxiety and depression I learned about. I learned to discount any talk of being "laid aside." What might seem to be useless days and hours can become fruitful and effective. Instead of being laid aside, the person who trusts God is actually still in the mainstream. God may be switching the mainstream for a while, but the patient is there for a purpose. And usefulness may still be experienced at such times.

I had often decried the lack of time my schedule allowed for prayer. My personal interest in missions as board chairman of Greater Europe Mission and acting medical director for Medical Assistance Programs, my concern for all my patients, and other prayer interests began to receive some of the time and attention I had longed to give them.

Sometimes I was just too sick or exhausted to pray. "Lord," I said at such times, "I'm just too tired to pray tonight. You just pray through me if You want to; I'm too tired even to make the effort."

Too, I had wanted to spend more time reading the Bible. I believe its claim that it is "profitable for teaching, for reproof, for correction, for training in righteousness." Like Billy Graham's father-in-law, the late Dr. L. Nelson Bell, I heartily recommend and prescribe one of the thirty-one chapters of Proverbs for each day of the month. And now I had the time.

But you can become saturated—even with reading the Word of God. You should not feel guilty about this, however. Simply shift gears and read some other type of literature: adventure, history, sports, mystery, romance.

As a busy professional man, I've often wanted more time to spend with my wife and children. Here was my golden opportunity, and what a rich experience to become reacquainted with them.

Depending on the nature of our illness, of course, there are many things we can do to make the time eminently worthwhile. I would not have believed the wide variety of pastimes in which one can engage while on a sickbed or while recuperating, except that I had about seventy days of my own to try to fill profitably.

When my strength began to return, I walked the few short blocks to the city library. There I studied subjects I knew little about: Jewish history, for example. I read many books, kept three-by-five file cards, and learned fascinating aspects of the subject, some quite important in relation to my work as a physician. It was a Jew, Jonas Salk, who produced the injectable polio vaccine. It was another Jew, Albert Sabin, who produced the oral vaccine for polio. For centuries, Europe used medical textbooks written by Jews. On and on it went. Valuable historical data became second nature to me.

I realized that many bedridden people today can use their minds to help others (writers, editors, ministers) by researching specific topics. Someone can pick up books at the library for them, and the research can begin. By avoiding deadlines, the patient is eased from any pressure that might otherwise be present. My own pastor concurred in the idea: bedridden members could research subjects he wanted to talk about in coming months. One invalid I know keeps books for a nursing home. The possibilities are limitless.

A marketing consultant I know has five secretaries, one of whom does nothing but read magazines and clip them for resource material. That same kind of service could be provided by bedridden people for editors, pastors and other Christian leaders.

A boy in our neighborhood, a high school senior, spent many hours building up card files of affirmative and negative arguments for debates. A shut-in member of a congregation could do something similar for his pastor.

By exercising my mind deliberately and continuously, it soon ran over with ideas, many of which I didn't have time to explore. I visualized a L'Abri-like place in a wooded scene where eminent retired professors and their spouses might live in small homes. Students might come for one quarter of their training to sit at the feet of these distinguished educators—the old Oxford idea of a tutorial system. Meetings would be informal, with only a few lectures scheduled during a week. Mature students in contact with great thinkers might accomplish a great deal in many ways.

And that is only typical of other ideas that came to mind as I had time and *took* time to think about many things. The mind's creative processes often function best at such times and under such circumstances.

Correspondence courses—in Bible, in writing, in many other subjects—provide a very worthwhile pastime for the sick person.

I learned anew that writing itself is a valuable ministry—letters of blessing, of inspiration, of testimony, of encouragement; articles for magazines; notes of appreciation; letters to editors.

Though I have not tried it in any organized or disciplined way, many people use the telephone as a very effective witnessing instrument—an evangelistic tool. An introductory explanation about one's physical disability often assures a listening ear. And since "the word of God is living and active and sharper than any two-edged sword," the weight of its message quite likely will lodge and bear fruit in many needy hearts.

I learned of things others do as circumstances

permit: make toys, flower arrangements, handcrafts, posters, do various types of sewing.

Surely, as I found, the radio provides a convenient medium for fruitful diversion, not only from the blessing of listening to and absorbing a message but also by responding to such programs and messages with letters of encouragement both to speakers and to station personnel, as well as to persons in need whose plight has been told via the airwaves. Perhaps we can help radio stations and Christian organizations from time to time by stuffing envelopes, addressing and stamping them—or by mailing out books and pamphlets for them.

All of this can happen, yet without feeling pressured. In fact, I learned to laugh at the clock. "Clock," I would say in mock disdain, "I don't have to pay any attention to you today." And for a busy physician, that was a priceless luxury, even at the cost of my health for a period.

The sky is the limit—depending, of course, on the physical condition of the individual patient. Even if confined to a hospital, we may have opportunity to witness to other patients.

At the very least, one need not be idle. We surely can *pray*—and we know we are heard. And this subject is so important, in fact, that you'll find a whole chapter about it later.

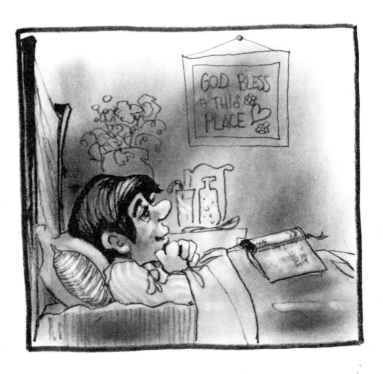

making the best of it

Every physical problem, whether medical or surgical, is a strain, and my situation certainly was no exception. My emotional reaction to hepatitis played an important part in my recovery, and it will be the same with you.

Even a broken leg produces strong emotional reactions: the strain of having to wear a cast, the pressure of bills that result, the forced inactivity, etc. Many of these problems are primarily psychological, and I have found the Bible to be the best possible textbook on psychology.

In an obvious oversimplification, I have discovered that there are only two types of problems in life: (1) those we can cope with, and (2) those we can't cope with. I found it difficult to cope with limited activity, realizing it might limit my income. But such problems for a mature Christian become God's problems, and surely none of them are too big for Him to handle.

Something can be learned from everything God allows to happen in our lives—valuable lessons to be gained no other way. "Lord, enable me to be patient through all of this," I remember praying. And this did come about, but only because of the strain and pressure that are a natural part of such situations.

In a variety of ways too numerous to mention, sick and suffering people have vowed to make the best of their condition and in so doing have found a joy and victory they would otherwise have missed.

One of these was a former patient of mine, Erwin (Zeke) Rudolph, twenty-one-year-old son of Dr. Erwin Paul Rudolph, Wheaton College professor who told his story in the book *Goodby, My Son*.

Though Zeke fought a losing battle with multiple sclerosis, he won a spiritual battle that affected the lives of scores, then hundreds, of people as Dr. Rudolph shared his thrilling story. Some of Zeke's writings in his last days on earth reveal his profound thinking and personal adjustment to a situation over which he had no control.

Although I am only twenty-one and have experienced only a portion of the average lifespan, I feel a definite sensitivity to the gigantic importance of finding the ultimate meaning to life. Death is as much a part of life as living. No one can escape it. Fear of it is only human, but I have found an assurance that truly overcomes this fear. It is a true belief in a supernatural God.

This was not a blind leap, nor was it logical reasoning totally, but an overcoming feeling brought on by something much greater than myself....Meaning cannot be found inwardly in a humanistic manner, but it seems to me that it has to be poured in outwardly. Each individual

44

has to open himself up and unlock his soul, using more than his mind to find meaning.

Meaning for me has come unhypocritically and honestly through a personal relationship with the God-man, Jesus Christ. To me, He is Being itself. I do not consider this mere emotion, but a reality. Christ's teachings have brought meaning to my life, not in a legalistic or moral way, but through an inspired feeling and assurance of their validity.

In a very real sense, God had prepared Zeke Rudolph for his grand entrance to a heavenly home. He will do the same for any of His children at the appropriate time in their lives. As someone has well said, "God does not give dying grace until one is dying," and in the same way He will give grace for whatever degree of physical disability or sickness one may have.

The Apostle Paul, though not given divine deliverance from his "thorn in the flesh," heard God say, "My grace is sufficient for you . . ."— and that is real victory. Such victory comes often under the most unusual circumstances.

Take the case of Miss Gray Pifer, for example, as told in James R. Adair's book *God's Power Within*. Though blind, she felt she could have a profitable ministry as a speech motivationist with cerebral palsy children. Against seemingly impossible odds, she accomplished what no one else felt she could. She had truly learned to make the best of her situation.

At the Villa Rose Rehabilitation Center in Sebring, Florida, Miss Pifer found many ingenious ways to make up for the lack of her eyesight as she taught the handicapped children. Authorities had told her it was impossible for a blind person to cope with the problems of teaching a C.P. child, but she won high praise for her talent in teaching speech by use of music to the spastic children.

Many cerebral palsy victims find it difficult to utter a single sound. Gray, drawing on her musical experience, fashioned a given sound into an attractive little melody. Then she induced the patient to sing it. This exercise of the vocal cords gradually produced an ability to speak words—a giant step along the trail to normal living.

A college student sent to Villa Rose for special help said, "How wonderful to make a song or game out of it! If only someone had made it so simple for me when I was learning."

Gray Pifer had learned how to cope with her own physical handicap. Her attitude perhaps best can be summed up in the words of Richard Dunwoody following his heart attack: "When the suffering soul quits rebelling and murmuring, and reaches a calm, sweet carelessness, when it can inwardly smile at its own suffering, the quietness of eternity settles down into the whole being."

I found that true in my own experience. Unable to answer the many questions my own heart and mind had raised, I simply determined to make the best of the unhappy situation in every way possible. And my heavenly Father, who was watching me—and over me—all the time, responded to that determination with many ideas and diversions that could not have come solely from me.

Real sickness is never enjoyable, but our experience in and through it can lead to real joy. The choice is ours.

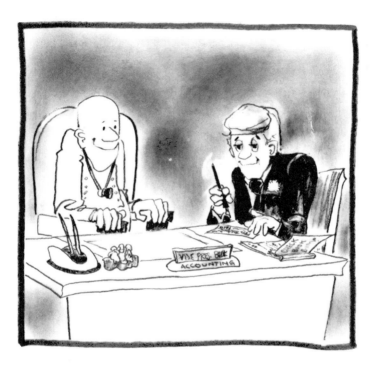

how to delight the doctor

By all means, at the first sign of illness or disability of any kind, we should take the matter to the Lord in prayer. To seek His help, His counsel, His direction is always right. Then, having done this, we should use the common sense He gives to accelerate our healing—for actually *all* healing comes from Him.

Doctors and medicines have been provided for our health and comfort. When the time comes to use them, we should be sure to use them wisely.

It is not at all inconsistent to place our confidence in the Lord while at the same time we look to one of His servants, the physician, for treatment.

Ideally, at the outset of a sickness or disability, we should begin by immediately praying, trusting God for the final healing—whether by instantaneous act or by progressive treatment and recovery. Having done this, we should commit the condition to our personal physician and work together with him to effect complete healing.

If this pattern is followed to the letter, we can properly begin too by thanking the Lord for healing *in His own good time,* with or without means. The general thrust of Scripture is that God wants us to prosper—in health and in every other way. We should act on that assumption, even though seeming exceptions to the rule do occur from time to time.

If we combine that act of trust and faith with the sacrifice of praise referred to earlier, we have an unbeatable combination. If we have doubts along the way, we should remember to "let the peace of Christ rule [or, *be the umpire*] in your hearts" to let us know if we are on the right track.

In my own experience, and certainly in that of countless thousands of others, God has used the therapy of sickness and diseases to teach important lessons. Our speed in learning is often the determining factor as to the length of our suffering.

Occasionally, however, God allows illness for the benefit of others. To the atheist or agnostic, one of the best demonstrations of God is to see a child of His under stress. The difference in the life of the believer shows up best under pressure.

One of life's great mysteries is the matter of pain and suffering. In my extended illness I gained a new insight into the subject. For me, the mystery is beginning to unravel, if only a few threads. A loving mother or father, eager to see a child develop his talent and become more proficient in playing the piano, may cause the child to "suffer" through endless practice. But the suffering is for a purpose: for the good of the child. Isn't it logical that a loving heavenly Father wants His children to grow, to develop their talents, to learn? My own case proved that pain and suffering was the best way He could teach me, so I reveled in His school of learning.

As we proceed through hours and days of illness, we must be sure to maintain a thoroughly open relationship with our physician. If he is to help us to the utmost of his ability, he must have our complete confidence. And we can trust him for complete secrecy about all that concerns us.

Let me stress the importance of following your doctor's orders to the letter. If for any reason you do not feel that his remedy or treatment is helping you, by all means let him know before you take it upon yourself to follow another course of action.

In my case, I discussed my condition with my colleague, who very graciously let me stay home instead of going to the hospital, even though he would have preferred the latter. Like most good doctors, he did not reject me because I didn't completely follow his advice. When he suggested I needed to keep my weight up, and that proteins would provide the most help, I began to nibble on food—mostly cheese—some eight or ten times a day, and occasionally during the night hours.

For a doctor, it is especially hard to accept the fact that there is no known medicine for a certain disease, particularly in a day of miracle cures through modern medicine. I had to learn patience and, of course, am still learning it, not unlike the man who prayed, "Lord, give me patience and give it to me in a hurry."

It is this same struggle with patience that I find prevalent among many of the college students I treat in my part-time work at the health center of Wheaton College. I remind students often that the decision is up to them; it is simply a matter of priorities. "If you want to get well sooner," I tell them, "you will find that staying in bed will help you." A valuable part of a young person's maturing is to see and understand this.

Even more important than physical rest, in a sense, is the matter of emotional rest. If fussing and fuming accompanies your rest, you might as well forget it. Stress promotes and aggravates illness. The body heals much faster when a person is tranquil.

Along with rest and tranquility is another important consideration perhaps not fully realized by many. Have you ever thought seriously about praying for your doctor? Many of them lead extremely busy lives, almost totally exhausting at times. They have their personal needs just as you do: family problems, physical concerns, severe busyness, and all that you might imagine would go along with the life of a modern physician.

As in other professions, they must bear the brunt of an unfavorable reputation brought about by the excesses and extravagances of a few. Each one should be judged on his own merit and not by the loose terms bandied about by the ill-informed or misinformed. Once you have settled on your own personal or family physician, by all means show complete confidence in him as he proceeds with your case.

Even as the Apostle Paul refers to Luke as the "beloved physician," may it be true that we can consider our own personal or family doctor in such a light. The Great Physician Himself desires that we be in good health; it is the normal thing. May it be our prayer and desire that all of His children experience that degree of health which He decrees for us.

To sum up: let's have confidence in the Lord first, then in our doctor. Let's pray for him, even as we do for others.

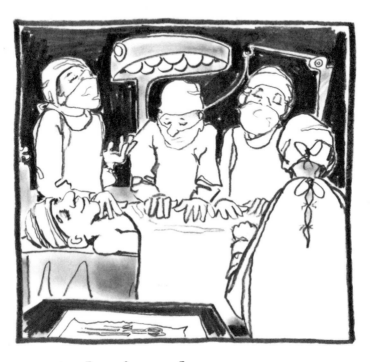

today's only sure cure

So-called miracle medicines have been a part of the profession as long as I can remember. And with due respect for them all, many of which do provide remarkable degrees of healing, I maintain there is only one sure cure in the whole field of medicine. If you guessed *prayer*, you have hit the nail on the head. Let me try to illustrate.

Prayer does not have to be spoken to be effective. In my own case, I have experienced times when I was too tired and exhausted to pray. But the Lord looks on the heart, and He can hear its inner voice most clearly. We should never feel we have reached the point of inability to pray.

Prayer accomplishes at least one other great benefit: it helps to remove hindrances to the victorious Christian life, and thus paves the way for the desired healing. Many times I have seen patients who have told of opening up their lives before the Lord in prayer and asking Him to purify, to cleanse and reveal anything that might be standing in the way of complete health and victory in their lives.

If somehow we could see and understand that there is no such thing as purposeless pain in God's economy, our suffering might take on a whole new light. It would still hurt, but the pain would be mitigated by the satisfying assurance that God never acts out of whim or caprice.

My parents set an early example for me that I will never forget. As a lad of seven in the second grade, I had an infected ear that quickly became mastoiditis. The doctor explained to my parents that an abscess was forming and I should be taken to a specialist.

Though both my mother and father were still in school, they ran a small dry-cleaning establishment. On hearing the word from the doctor, they closed up the plant and spent an entire day in fasting and prayer. By the next morning, without any medicine, the infection had localized. After drainage, it healed—and I suffered no hearing loss.

In this case, I believe, the Lord used the doctor and a natural sequence of events to speed up my healing. My father told me later he had committed my life to the Lord in a specific way at that time.

In my experience, the results of earnest intercession have been as varied as they have been rewarding. I know there are times when the miraculous—instantaneous healing—takes place. I do not know why this takes place so seldom, nor do I believe it necessarily implies a lack of faith on the part of the seeker when the miracle does not occur.

I am reminded of Charles Spurgeon's rejoinder to a student who wondered at some of God's mysteries: "You must expect to let God know some things which you do not understand."

Miracles occur most often, it seems, when finite man reaches the limit of his ability to help. "Man's extremity is God's opportunity," and this is never more true than in the realm of health and healing.

You have heard it said, and rightly so: "God's timing is always perfect." Is it any less a miracle when God chooses to heal progressively rather than instantaneously? Who knows the divine mystique that sees the need for greater or lesser periods of seasoning before the healing is complete? Who knows what one person's illness is accomplishing in other hearts and lives, which helps determine the exact time when healing comes?

As a general rule, in my experience, at least, healing comes over a period of time and is dependent on several important factors: mental and spiritual attitude of the patient, his degree of compliance with the doctor's wishes, the extent of the person's illness, and others. All other things being equal, the physician usually can discern the approximate period of time that an illness will require before recovery takes place.

Perhaps a third general classification, involving a fewer number of people, has to do with those to whom healing never comes. In each of these three major areas, prayer plays a vital part—and prayer is just as really answered here as in the other two. Is it not true in your experience, as it has been in mine, that spiritual accomplishments often are more plentiful and pronounced in the lives of the sick and suffering than in any others?

Even as the deaths of martyrs in yesteryear, and today as well, command the sacrificial response of untold thousands of young and old alike, so the saintlike suffering of God's army of the sick today quite often brings about a similar response and challenges thousands of lives. Both directly and indirectly, the sick person has the potential for great spiritual benefit to be effected in the lives of others as they watch his behavior under pressure.

Prayer is the leavening, softening, purifying ingredient that makes of illness a benediction that can change thousands of lives in the process. No other activity or remedy or prescription or therapy can accomplish one fraction of the eternal good that will result from prayer. It is not a magic mumbo jumbo of the abracadabra type, but rather a personal confrontation with the Creator of the universe and a glorious conversation with one who loves us.

Let me encourage you, in health and in sickness, to spend time with Him. By all means, thank Him when you are in good health. As my good friend Ray Knighton, president of Medical Assistance Programs, puts into daily practice, begin every day by thanking God for the degree of health you have. It will do wonders for you, whatever your condition might happen to be at any particular time.

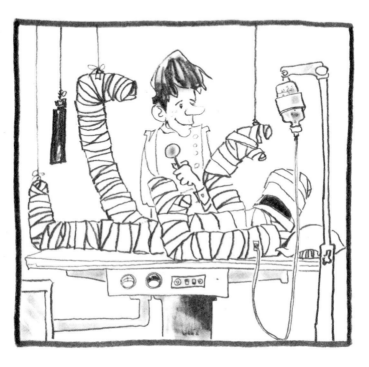

when you can't lick 'em . . .

Death and taxes historically have been listed among the inevitables that cloud man's life. Add sickness, suffering, and sorrow to the list, as I have had to do, and you will not be far wrong. But such knowledge should not lead to despair or discouragement, but rather to sober reflection and careful preparation.

Richard Dunwoody has some interesting mathematics for us to consider:

> Defeat plus grace equals victory; loss plus grace equals gain. These are advanced spiritual algebraic equations. Paul, in speaking of the Macedonian Christians, gave us the greatest mathematical equation in the world: "For in the midst of an ordeal of severe tribulation, their abundance of joy, and their depth of poverty (together) have overflowed in a wealth of lavish generosity on their part" (II Cor. 8:2 ANT). Severe tribulation plus joy plus poverty equal lavish generosity! What an equation! Christ, and His grace, are the least common denominator that reduces all fractions and parts into wholes and completions. Christ is better with His cross than the world with its crown.

Surely, you and I should find some genuine

consolation in the certain knowledge that sickness, sorrow, and suffering are the common lot of all mankind. Granted, there are varying degrees of severity in each of these areas; nevertheless, we experience a real kinship in knowing we are not alone. Since it is inevitable, our approach to sickness will certainly have an effect on its severity, its length or duration, and the lessons learned from it.

Perhaps you are now in the throes of a serious bout of illness, and you have no time to consider any kind of preparation for such sickness. The fact remains there are still positive steps you can take:

(1) Let your best friends, those who pray, know you have a physical need and that you will appreciate their prayer interest. In the same way that Billy Graham receives divine power for his evangelistic ministry through the worldwide intercession of concerned friends, so you will be strengthened by the spiritual impact of prayer.

In this matter of prayer, never feel that your condition is too trivial or too serious for intercessory intervention. "You do not have because you do not ask" (James 4:2). Let's not have that said of us.

We should take advantage of every available means for help. If your church practices the suggestion of James to call for the elders and anoint with oil in the name of the Lord, that step of faith should be followed. In so doing, you are committing your situation to the one who created you, and surely you can be in no better hands. Let's expect Him to help, with or without means, instantaneously or progressively. The decision is His.

(2) Having prayed and committed our condition to Him, let's look for every way possible to use our time wisely—in the numerous ways suggested earlier, and others that will come to our minds.

(3) Insofar as possible, let's become prayerfully concerned and involved in the problems of others. In an amazing way, this will serve to soften our own trials. This can be done in a variety of ways, dependent upon our own condition and circumstances.

(4) Let's keep up our reading in the Word of God and in related books with spiritual help and warmth. If our condition makes this impossible, we should find a friend who will read to us. Let's make known our requests—not only to the Lord but also to those of our friends and loved ones who want to help us.

(5) Let's be as honest with the Lord as we know how to be. We should not pretend with Him; He knows us better than anyone else.

(6) Let's not confuse illness with punishment; the two rarely, if ever, go together. True, God's conditioning process often involves tempering, but this should never be confused with punishment. To be conformed to His image should be our supreme goal in life; this cannot be

accomplished aside from the fiery furnace of suffering.

May our goal truly be expressed in the words of Scripture: "That with all boldness, Christ shall . . . be exalted in my body, whether by life or by death" (Philippians 1:20).

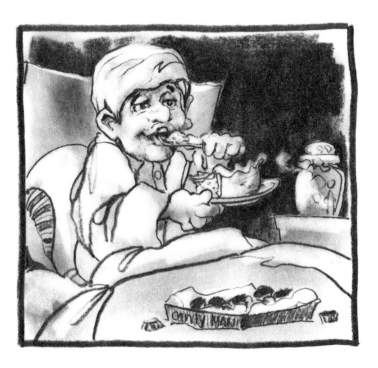

how to stay sweet
though sick

One verse in particular which helped me was Hebrews 12:15—"See to it that no one comes short of the grace of God; that no root of bitterness springing up cause trouble, and by it many be defiled."

Whenever the subject of bitterness is mentioned in the New Testament, it refers to something pointed, sharp, and pungent. Matthew 26:75 tells about Peter weeping bitterly; he had been stricken in his conscience. A religious quack is described in Acts 8:23 as being "in the gall of bitterness" when he tried to appear godly and spiritual.

Hebrews 12:15 talks about a *root,* and certainly a bitter root can bear nothing but bitter fruit. Ordinarily, the person hurt most by the sin of bitterness is the one who is guilty of committing it, though of course it will affect others as well. Most serious, perhaps, is the fact that the bitter person has not truly learned how to forgive, and as a result he poisons all that he touches.

When the Apostle Paul begins to talk about things the Christian should avoid at all costs, we note his first target. "Let all *bitterness* and wrath and anger and clamor and slander be put away from you, along with all malice. And be kind to one another, tender-hearted, forgiving each other, just as God in Christ also has forgiven you."

You and I soon discover that the awful effect of bitterness is twofold. First, a bitter person leaves himself wide open to all kinds of stress and strain that lead to various kinds of illness. Surely it is not worth the "luxury" of ill feelings when they lead to physical disturbances.

Second, one who is bitter toward God—whether expressed or not, and possibly not even fully realized—often hinders the healing process in his own body. Simple logic obviates against the likelihood of divine intervention in our physical condition where fellowship has been threatened, if not completely broken.

What can we do about the spiritual and physical impasse that results from bitterness? Several things come immediately to mind. First, let's be honest enough before God and before men to admit that a root of bitterness exists— if it does. This may take some careful self-examination, for we may successfully hide such a feeling for years, even from ourselves. But it is well worth the effort to ferret it out so that deliverance might be sought and obtained.

Then, we will find a simple yet practical way to overcome such bitterness. It is twofold in its implementation. If the feeling is primarily against God because of events that have happened in our lives, our only remedy is praise—true thanksgiving to God for His many blessings, until the feeling becomes fact as we realize that He has indeed blessed us richly.

If our feeling of bitterness is against another human being, at least one way of victory is guaranteed. We should begin to pray earnestly for the person involved, asking God to bless him or her abundantly and make him all he should be. Not only will such prayers be gloriously answered, but a strange and dynamic thing will also take place: our feelings of bitterness magically turn to thoughts of concern and love. The root of bitterness is completely pulled up and out.

Lest this whole exercise seem blown out of proportion, let me stress the importance of mental and spiritual health before we can expect to enjoy physical health. Bitterness may seem like a harmless luxury to some, but to the God who requires love from His children, it is a heinous sin and must be dealt with accordingly.

Perhaps it would be helpful if we seek to determine why bitterness is so wrong. Basically, it reveals a lack of faith—particularly as it relates to our feeling toward God. The heinousness of bitterness must be realized, but it must never be considered outside the scope of God's forgiveness. The blessed truth remains: "If we confess our sins, he is faithful and righteous to forgive us our sins and to cleanse us from all unrighteousness."

Concerning a bitter feeling toward another human: if nothing else, the sin comes from disobedience to God, who commands us to love one another. Either way, confession, repentance, and forgiveness are necessary before we find the road to victory.

In the words of Scripture, I encourage you to "put away bitterness." It's the sure way to good health.

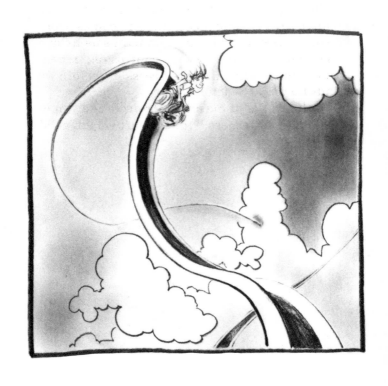

the road to perfect peace

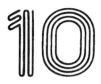

In my own extended illness, I learned of some things more important than good health—as wonderful and glorious as that is. Strangely enough, I felt no compulsion to pray for my own healing, so convinced was I that God had me in His school of suffering for good reasons. He would release me in His own good time. Meanwhile, I wanted to learn . . . to grow . . . to earn His "Well-done."

By no means did His ten-week course answer all my questions of sickness, suffering, and pain. But it did provide some of the answers, and for me it meant a giant step forward in my desire to serve others.

One key lesson I learned: man's wisdom can't hold a candle to the Word of God, particularly when His Holy Spirit becomes our Teacher as we read and study His Word. The same applies with this volume you are now reading: only as it shares experiences of believers or quotes, interprets, and reflects the Word and the will of God will it have value for you. Let's ask Him to teach us as we review these truths.

Perhaps we need to be reminded that we serve a loving God who not only controls the universe but who also loves every individual as personally as if you and I had been the only ones who ever lived. If His love is that real and that personal—and surely it is—what do we have to fear from whatever He permits to happen in our lives?

One cause of sickness I have not mentioned thus far; hence this brief reminder. Carelessness and abuse of our own bodies can lead to illnesses of various kinds. Health can come only when we obey the physical laws that lead to a healthy condition.

If proof were needed that God is interested in our bodies being healthy, we need only remember that they are called the temple of the Holy Spirit; also, how His Son, Jesus Christ, went about healing and doing good when He was here on earth. And the whole context of Scripture bears out the idea that He wants us to be in good health.

Up to this point, I have assumed that you are a believer in the Lord Jesus Christ, one who has trusted Him personally for salvation. Perhaps this is a warranted assumption, but is too important an issue to pass over lightly. Quite logically, we cannot expect help from a kind heavenly Father if we have not truly and personally recognized Him in that capacity.

If you are interested in a further study of the subject of salvation or conversion, let me encourage you to read the Gospel of John and follow its suggestions carefully. They will surely lead you to personal faith in Christ as they have literally millions of others in the past. Only then can you expectantly ask and receive help from Him for physical and other needs that concern your life.

Let's keep in mind that God does not always heal. For reasons known only to Him, sickness sometimes remains for extended periods. The challenge then is to search our own heart and life for reasons, and lacking them, to learn to adjust. It may seem like a tough way to proceed, but again it often provides the only road to personal victory.

God's loving purpose for your life may not be fully revealed this side of heaven, but you have to know and believe that He truly has your best interest at heart. At times, we will say with the Apostle Paul, "Most gladly, therefore, I will rather boast about my weaknesses, that the power of Christ may dwell in me" (2 Corinthians 12:9).

None of us ever really wants to be sick, even though the Word talks about "the fellowship of His sufferings" as something to be desired. Whatever that means, we know that growth in grace often is preceded and/or accompanied by sickness and suffering. Though the cost may seem high, surely it results in our becoming more Christlike.

When Matthew 6:33 speaks of seeking first the Kingdom of God, it almost at times necessitates the discipline of suffering, without which most of us would never truly concentrate on things above to the exclusion of the material.

Sometimes empathy and sympathy are lacking in our dealings with others because we have not known adversity for a long time. To learn that lesson, sickness is often necessary. Many of us forget to look up until we are flat on our backs.

Sickness can be a blessing—especially if we are open before God to learn whatever lesson He might be trying to teach us at the time. Many a sickroom has become a workroom or a pulpit. Blind Fanny Crosby wrote hundreds of poems and hymns. It may be that your service for the Lord can be accomplished more effectively from a sickbed. That requires spiritual discernment and discipline of the highest order. We can ask and expect such from God.

And finally, if you ever desire the sympathy and fellowship of another sufferer, turn to the Psalms. They will encourage and cheer you as you find the Psalmist's questions—and answers—to the problem of sickness.

My ten weeks with hepatitis, a valuable spiritual experience for me, left me physically weak, so that I had to resume my practice on a part-time basis. But it was not many weeks before I was back in full swing.

Meanwhile, I believe the lessons learned have made me a better Christian, a better husband, a better father, and a better doctor. Could I ask for anything more?